# 6

## MINUTE
## MORNING

### ARMS

# 6 MINUTE MORNING
## ARMS

LUCY WYNDHAM-READ

Bath · New York · Singapore · Hong Kong · Cologne · Delhi · Melbourne

First published by Parragon in 2009

Parragon
Queen Street House
4 Queen Street
Bath BA1 1HE, UK

ISBN: 978-1-4075-8122-4

Printed in Malaysia
Created and produced by Ivy Contract
Design: JC Lanaway
Photography: Ian Parsons
Hair and Makeup: Sarah El Hini
Model: Willow Boswell-Wright

The views expressed in this book are those of the author, but they are general views
only, and readers are urged to consult a relevant and qualified specialist for individual
advice in particular situations. Parragon hereby excludes all liability to the extent
permitted by law for any errors or omissions in this book and for any loss, damage,
or expense (whether direct or indirect) suffered by a third party relying on any
information contained in this book.

Ivy Contract would like to thank iStock/Michael Tupy for permission to reproduce
copyright material on pages 6–7.

Thanks to Inter Sport of Lewes in the UK for providing props for photography.

**Caution**
Please check with your doctor/therapist before attempting this workout,
particularly if you have an injury, are pregnant, or have just had a baby. It is
recommended that new mothers wait at least six weeks postpartum before
participating in exercise (12 weeks if it was a Cesarean birth). If you feel any pain or
discomfort at any point, please stop exercising immediately and seek medical advice.

# CONTENTS

# INTRODUCTION

The arms and upper body is an area that is often overlooked when undertaking exercise routines. This can result in the muscles becoming weak and saggy, which may lead to poor posture and even health problems.

By exercising your arms and upper body, you can achieve an incredibly toned and svelte shape. Exercising will also help to lift your bust naturally, banish any wobble from your arms, shape and tone your shoulders, define your back, and increase your upper-body strength.

Working on your upper body also helps to realign your muscles, which will enhance your posture and immediately make you look slimmer and more confident.

**Clothing**
*Wear clothes that you can remove in layers, made from a comfortable and breathable fabric.*

Your arms and upper body contain some major muscle groups, so working on this area will naturally raise your metabolic rate. As well as toning and increasing your strength, you will also be "melting away" any excess calories by working harder.

The easy-to-follow exercises within this book have been specially designed to target all the areas of the upper body, including the back of the upper arms, the shoulders, the bust, and the back. In as little as 6 minutes a day, you can have a beautifully toned upper body that you can show off with confidence, instead of hiding it under long-sleeved shirts and sweaters!

## How to use this book

Simply choose six of the exercises from the book. Always start with the warm-up and stretches, then finish off with the cooldown routines. Try to follow the exercises on a daily basis. There is a wide selection to choose from to keep your training varied and maintain your motivation.

If you look at the two-week plan (see page 44), you will see how to fit the warm-up and the exercises into 6 minutes. We have made it easy for you to see what you should be doing on each day.

## What you need

Some of the exercises require hand weights. These come in different sizes; you can lift slightly heavier ones as you increase your upper-body fitness. We have used 2 pound (purple) and 5 pound (blue) weights. Women can use either weight for any of the exercises, or no weight at all if you prefer. If you don't have any weights, small plastic milk cartons filled with either rice grains or sand are a great alternative. It is a good idea to perform your exercises in front of a mirror so you can assess your technique. Always make sure the room is well ventilated and well lit, and that you have enough room to stretch your arms fully upward and out to the side.

It is best to wear layers of breathable, comfortable fabric. It's also worth having a clock visible, with a second hand, so you can time yourself for each exercise. You will need a chair for a couple of the exercises, as well as a mat or a towel for the floor exercises.

## What time of the day to exercise

If you have enough time, doing these exercises in the morning is a great way to kick-start your day because this will speed up your metabolic rate and you will burn off more calories. You will also feel virtuous for the rest of the day, knowing that you have done your exercises! But the great thing with a 6-minute workout is that you should always be able to find time in the day to squeeze it in.

## Getting started

First, use the two-week planner at the back of the book to get started. If you want to develop your own two-week plan later on, you can. After warming up, choose six of the 30-second exercises, and repeat them so you are working for 6 minutes in total.

## The results of toning

Some women worry that if they do toning exercises for their upper body, they will become bulky. This is simply not true—women do not have enough testosterone to build large muscles. You would have to be lifting heavy weights and following a strict strength-training workout!

**Equipment**
*The basic equipment you need to perform the exercises are a mat, weights, and a sturdy chair.*

This exercise program is designed to create long, lean, defined muscles rather than muscle bulk. For men using this book, it is recommended to use weights with all the arm exercises. The reason for this is that men tend to have more upper-body strength than women, and it is important for every exercise to feel challenging. By using the hand weights, you can be sure that your workout is at the right intensity.

### Improving your upper body area

Achieving a supertoned body requires a combination of two forms of exercise: the first is toning, as described in this book, and the other is aerobic. The aerobic form of activity will help to burn off any excess body fat, as well as improve your cardiovascular health. You should also remember the importance of eating sensibly, because too many calories in your diet may increase your level of body fat.

### About your muscles

To tone and shape your upper body, it is helpful to have a clear understanding of the names and positions of the muscles of the upper body so you know which ones to focus on if you want to tackle any problem areas. It's important to keep the workout balanced by training all the muscles.

### Shoulders

The muscles that form your shoulders are known as the deltoids and consist of three sections, or heads. Each of these sections has different actions:

• The anterior (front) originates at the collarbone and moves your arms up and forward, as well as rotating inward.
• The lateral (side) head works primarily to lift your arms to the side and assist the anterior and posterior heads in their movements.
• The posterior (back) head attaches to your shoulder blade and moves your arms to the rear, as well as rotating them outward.

### Chest

The pectoralis major is a large, fan-shaped muscle that has several attachments. One portion fastens to the middle and inner parts of your collarbone, working with the front of your shoulder to move your arms in front and above, and to rotate them inward. The other part attaches to your breastbone and ribs—this muscle is activated by moving your arms only in a downward or forward movement of both arms.

## Upper arms

The biceps is the muscle that runs down the front of your upper arm. It allows you to flex your elbow and rotate your forearm so that your palms can face down. This muscle is attached to the shoulder joint and your elbow joint.

The muscle at the back of the upper arm is called the triceps. It is attached to the shoulder and the elbow, and it is activated by straightening the arm. This muscle can easily lose its tone, resulting in flabby-looking upper arms.

## Middle and lower back

The latissimus dorsi is the largest muscle in the upper body and covers the middle and lower back. This muscle is responsible for the downward movements of the upper arm and the inward rotation of your shoulders.

## Measure your progress

If you exercise regularly, you will soon see results, so a great way to keep motivated is to measure your progress. There are two ways of doing this.

First, try measuring your arms. Using your right arm, place a tape measure around the upper part of the arm, approximately a hand's distance down from your shoulder. Do this every two weeks, making sure you always measure in the same spot. You should notice the measurement becomes less as the muscle of the upper arms becomes more toned and you reduce excess fat.

Secondly, to see how much you have increased your upper-body fitness, try performing a push-up using the correct technique (see page 37), and see how many you can comfortably manage. Your performance should quickly improve.

## Push-ups

Make a note of the number of push-ups you do. You should find that push-ups become easier the more you do and you can perform more each time.

# WARMING UP

It is always essential to warm up before undertaking any form of exercise. Without an effective warm-up, you are likely to injure yourself while working out and you will be unable to perform your exercises efficiently.

Warming up naturally increases your core body temperature, which then warms up the muscles and makes them more pliable. It also increases the fluid in your joints, which enables you to be more flexible. Even though your toning exercises take only 6 minutes, you still need to warm up because injuries can occur at any time.

## Marching on the spot

This is a very easy and safe way to gently start warming up your body. Stand with good posture, by having your feet hips' width apart, knees slightly bent, abdomen pulled in, and shoulders pulled back. Starting from this position ensures that you are exercising in a safe manner. Begin marching on the spot. Be sure to keep your upper body straight and your abdominal muscles pulled in. Aim to gradually lift your knees to hip height, then bend your arms and swing them back and forth as you would do if you were walking fast. Do this for 2 to 3 minutes until you feel fully warmed up. Alternatively, you can warm up by going for a brisk walk around the block or, if you are in a gym, by using the stationary bike or treadmill.

## Shoulder Rolls

These ensure that you have fully warmed the shoulders and chest, and the shoulder joint is properly mobilized.

**1** Stand with good posture, and check that your feet are slightly wider than hips' width apart.

**2** Make sure your knees are slightly bent and that your abdominal muscles are pulled in tight toward your spine.

**3** Very slowly and gently, start to rotate through your shoulders by lifting your shoulders up, then behind. Each time, increase this movement and aim to make the circles bigger.

**4** Repeat the exercise 10 times.

## Arm Swing

This will increase the flexibility of your chest muscles and help to loosen your upper back.

**1** Stand with good posture, knees slightly bent and abdominal muscles pulled in.

**2** Lift both arms out to either side of your body.

**3** In a slow and controlled motion, bring both arms in front so they cross over, then back out to either side.

**4** Be sure to keep your abdominal muscles pulled in to maintain good posture throughout.

**5** Repeat the exercise 10 times.

### Stretches

Once you have warmed up, it is also important to stretch your muscles before you start the exercises. You should also do this at the end of your exercises when you cooldown.

### The benefits of stretching are:

• It reduces the risk of injury during activity.
• It helps prevent postexercise soreness.
• It improves your flexibility and range of movement.

### Deltoid Stretch

**1** Stand with good posture, extend one arm out in front of you, and cross it in front of the midline of your body.

**2** Keep both shoulders facing forward. Support the stretching arm on the fleshy part of the forearm.

**3** Hold this stretch on each arm for 10 seconds.

**BE AWARE**
Breathe normally when practicing abdominal hollowing; do not take a deep breath when trying to flatten your abdomen. If your rib cage rises during the movement, you have taken a deep breath.

2

## Triceps Stretch

**1** Stand with good posture, lift one arm above your head, and drop the palm of the hand behind the head between the shoulder blades.

**2** Lift the other arm, and support the stretching arm on the soft, fleshy part of the upper arm or just above the elbow.

**3** Hold this stretch on each arm for 10 seconds.

## Chest Stretch

If you spend a lot of time using a computer, your shoulders tend to draw in and rise upward. The chest stretch is good for counteracting this movement and helps to open up the shoulder and chest area.

**1** Stand with good posture, with your feet slightly apart.

**2** Clasp your hands together behind your back, and raise them until you feel the stretch in your chest.

**3** Keep your shoulders down as you hold onto your wrists.

**4** Hold this position for 10 seconds.

## Upper Back Stretch

This stretch is particularly good for improving your posture and releasing any tension in your back.

**1** Stand with good posture, with your feet slightly apart.

**2** Keep your knees slightly bent and your abdominal muscles pulled in.

**3** Take your arms out in front of you, and imagine you are hugging a big beach ball. You should feel a stretch across your upper back.

**4** Hold this position for 10 seconds.

2

3

## How to Exercise with Good Posture

Good posture is important all the time, but especially when exercising, because you need to be in the correct alignment for the appropriate muscles to be trained to get the best results. Imagine you have a glass sheet in front of you and behind you—this will help keep your body in alignment.

## Standing Exercises

**1** Stand with your feet just slightly wider than shoulders' width apart.

**2** Distribute your weight evenly through both feet.

**3** Extend up through your thighs, squeeze your buttocks in and under, and pull in your navel toward your spine.

**4** Stretch up through your spine, and let your shoulders drop down from the height of your ears.

**5** Contract the abdominal muscles by pulling your navel in toward your spine.

4

4

## Sitting Exercises

**1** Always ensure you use a sturdy chair for the sitting exercises.

**2** Place your feet hips' width apart, and make sure your heels are aligned directly under your knees.

**3** Sit upright and pull your navel in toward your spine—this will protect your back.

**4** Pull back your shoulders, and keep your chin parallel to the floor.

STANDING EXERCISES

The following exercises will all be performed standing up. This allows you to have a full range of movement. When lifting weights, always keep the movement slow and controlled. This not only works the muscles harder, but also prevents any injuries.

### Triceps Squeeze Back

This is an easy-to-perform standing exercise that will provide tone through the back of your upper arms, creating a long, toned triceps muscle and banishing any wobbly arms. The other great thing with this exercise is that it also stretches your chest muscles, which helps promote good posture.

**1** Stand with good posture and your knees slightly bent. Hold the weights, keeping your arms by your sides, with your palms facing backward.

**2** Lift your chest and pull your shoulders back.

**3** Lift both arms directly behind you, and feel this working through your triceps. Hold your arms at the highest point, then slowly lower back to the starting position.

**BE AWARE**

This is a small lift, so don't expect to raise your arms too high. Keep your knees slightly bent and your abdominal muscles pulled in tight.

1

3

**BE AWARE**
The arm that supports
your exercising arm
keeps the elbow in line
with your shoulder.

## Triceps Ponytail

This standing triceps exercise is one of
the best ways to tone flabby upper arms.

**1** Stand with good posture. Bend your
knees slightly, and pull in your abdominal
muscles. Hold a weight in your right hand,
then extend the right arm straight up and
support it with the other arm. Keep a good
posture and your abdominal muscles
pulled in.

**2** Now simply bend the elbow of
your extended arm so the weight is by
your upper back. Slowly straighten the arm
back up to the starting position. Do all your
repetitions on one arm, then repeat
on the other arm.

1

2

**BE AWARE**
To get your abdominal
muscles working, make
sure you keep your
abdomen pulled in tight
toward your spine.
Also, be sure not to
arch your back.

## Bell Pull

This exercise gives tone to your arms
through your biceps and triceps, as well
as toning your chest muscle. This is great
exercise for women because it helps lift
and tone the bust while giving the arms
a fabulous workout.

**1** Stand with good posture, knees slightly
bent and your feet hips' width apart.

**2** Lift your arms to shoulder height and
then bend at the elbows, so your arms
form an L shape. Press your arms together
and keep elbows at shoulder height.

**3** Take a deep breath in and then,
as you breathe out, gently lift your
arms a little bit higher, hold for a second,
then lower slowly again. Do all your
repetitions on one arm, then repeat
on the other arm.

2

3

## Standing Wall Push-Up

This exercise is a fantastic way to build upper-body strength, as well as provide tone through the back of your upper arm muscles and into your chest.

1 Stand at arms' length away from a wall, with your feet shoulders' width apart. Place your hands flat against the wall, with your arms stretched out in front of you and your fingers pointing to the ceiling.

2 Keeping your back straight and your head looking straight in front of you, slowly bend your arms at the elbows.

3 Aim to lower yourself a little way toward the wall, then push back to your starting position.

**BE AWARE**
Keep your elbows slightly bent while performing this to avoid locking your elbow joints.

**BE AWARE**
If you want to increase the level of difficulty, try moving your legs farther back. Also, keeping your abdominal muscles pulled in will help tone them at the same time.

## Shoulder Press

This will help to provide tone through your shoulders and triceps, as well as promote good upper-body posture.

1 Stand with good posture, knees slightly bent and abdomen pulled in. Hold a weight in each hand at shoulder height.

2 With your palms facing forward and keeping your head level, press the weights overhead, extending your elbows.

3 Bring the weights together as you press them, hold for a second, then slowly lower to the starting position.

### Upright Pull

This exercise will provide tone through your shoulders, biceps, and back, which will help you achieve a beautifully toned upper body.

**1** Stand with your feet shoulders' width apart and your knees slightly bent.

**2** Hold a weight in each hand, side by side and in front of you at thigh level, keeping your palms facing toward your thighs.

**3** Slowly bring the weights up toward your collarbone, until your elbows are about shoulder height. Keep your shoulders down and relaxed as you lift. If you find you are shrugging your shoulders up toward your ears, your weights may be too heavy.

**4** Slowly lower the weights to the starting position.

**BE AWARE**
Ensure you keep your weights close to your body as you lift and lower them.

2

**3** Slowly lift the weights out to the sides to shoulder level, keeping your elbows slightly bent. Keep your shoulders down and relaxed as you lift. If you find you are shrugging your shoulders up toward your ears, your weights may be too heavy.

**4** Slowly lower the weights back to the starting position.

**BE AWARE**
It's important to keep a slight bend in both arms as you lift them. Imagine both arms are pouring water from a pitcher; this helps to keep them slightly bent.

3

## Side Shoulder Raise

This exercise will help to define your shoulders—it is also good for improving flexibility throughout your shoulder joints and will give you good posture.

**1** Stand with your feet shoulders' width apart and your knees slightly bent.

**2** Hold the hand weights at your sides at thigh level.

### Turning Press

This is a great time-saving exercise because it targets several upper-body muscles at once, including your triceps, biceps, and shoulders.

1 Stand with your feet hips' width apart, upper body straight, knees slightly bent, and abdominal muscles pulled in.

2 Hold a weight in each hand with your palms facing directly in front of your shoulders and your elbows bent as if in a biceps curl (see page 35).

3 Straighten your elbows and lift the weights overhead, twisting the hands until the palms face out. Lower your arms and twist your palms to face inward again.

### Front Raises

This exercise will sculpt your shoulders and create tone and definition through the front of your arms.

1 Stand with good posture, your feet hips' width apart, and knees slightly bent.

2 Keep your abdominal muscles tight and chest relaxed.

3 Hold a weight in each hand with palms facing inward, weights by your thighs.

4 In a slow and controlled smooth move, lift both arms up forward and straight to shoulder height, then slowly lower both arms back to the starting position.

## Standing Long-Arm Palm Press

This exercise strengthens the front and the middle of your shoulders.

**1** Holding a weight in each hand, stand with good upright posture, knees slightly bent, abdominal muscles pulled in, and your feet shoulders' width apart.

**2** Lift both arms up and out to your sides so your wrists are in line with your shoulders and your palms facing upward.

**3** Now lift both arms up above your head, keeping the arms long. Try to bring your hands together to touch and hold for a second. Now very slowly lower your arms back to the starting position.

**BE AWARE**
When your arms are out to your sides, keep them parallel to your shoulders, not any higher or lower.

### Front Arm Toner (Hammer Curl)

This exercise will provide tone through the front of your upper arms and also works on strengthening your forearm muscles.

**1** Stand with your feet shoulders' width apart, knees slightly bent, elbows stiff, and abdominal muscles pulled in tight to promote good upper-body posture.

**2** With a weight in each hand, let both arms hang down long by the side of your body, fully straightened with your palms facing in toward your body.

**3** Simultaneously lift your weights upward, without moving your elbows, hold for a second, then slowly lower back to the starting position.

## Arm Opener

This exercise works by toning the biceps in your front upper arms. The exercise will firm the biceps, not bulk them out.

1 Stand with your feet shoulders' width apart, knees slightly bent, elbows stiff, and abdominal muscles pulled in tight to promote good upper-body posture.

2 Hold your arms by your side, with your elbows bent, and your arms in an L shape, a weight in each hand.

3 With your palms facing in toward each other, slowly open your forearms out to either side, while still keeping your elbows tucked into your sides. Hold for a second, then slowly return to the starting position.

**BE AWARE**
Keep this exercise slow and controlled. It is important to keep your elbows locked in tight to your side.

### Arm Circles

This easy-to-follow exercise will improve mobility and definition in your shoulders. You can increase the intensity by using hand weights or by simply creating bigger circles.

**1** Stand straight with your feet shoulders' width apart. Your arms should be straight out to the sides so that your body forms a T shape.

**2** Starting slowly, make small clockwise circular motions with both arms.

**3** Focus on keeping your knees slightly bent and your abdominal muscles pulled in throughout.

**BE AWARE**
The stronger you feel, the bigger you can make the circles.

3

## Chest Press

This exercise targets two muscles—your triceps and your chest muscle. This is a great exercise for women because it tightens the muscles that support your bust, giving you a good bust lift.

**1** Stand with good upright posture, knees slightly bent and your feet hips' width apart.

**2** Holding a weight in each hand, bend your arms so your hands are in front of your shoulders.

**3** Gently extend your arms straight out, keeping them at shoulder height.

**4** When your arms are fully extended, hold for a second. Slowly return your arms to the starting position.

**BE AWARE**

Focus on engaging your abdominal muscles by pulling your navel tight toward your spine. This helps protect your back.

### Arm Shaper (Boxing Arms)

This is a really fun exercise that will tone your arms, chest, and shoulders. When an exercise works several muscles at once, it increases the amount of calories you burn, both during and after the exercise.

**1** Stand up straight with your feet shoulders' width apart, abdominal muscles pulled in, and your knees slightly bent.

**2** Hold your hands level against your upper chest, with both your fists clenched and palms facing inward.

**3** Punch one arm forward under control, with your knuckles facing forward. Make sure your hands are held level and kept at shoulder height.

**4** Bring your hand back to the starting position, slowly and under control, then punch forward with the opposite arm.

**BE AWARE**
Keep your knees slightly bent and your abdomen pulled in. This will not only work your abdominal muscles, but also protect your back.

3

4

## Bust Lift

This exercise targets the chest muscle, which is responsible for supporting the bust. If this muscle is not exercised, it will become less supportive, which means the bust begins to droop. This is a great way of toning and giving yourself a bust lift.

1 Stand upright with good posture, knees slightly bent, feet hips' width apart, and abdominal muscles pulled in.

2 Extend your arms out in front of you at chest height, bend the elbows, and join your hands with the palms facing into each other.

3 Stay in this position, press into your palms and, holding this squeeze, slowly lift your palms a little bit higher. Hold for a second while still applying the squeeze, then slowly lower to the starting position, release the squeeze for a second, then reapply and lift.

**BE AWARE**
Keep this very slow and controlled. The more pressure you apply through the squeeze, the harder you work on lifting the bust.

# SITTING EXERCISES

For the following sitting exercises, always ensure you use a sturdy chair. These exercises will again target all the muscles in your upper body, helping to tone and define.

### Triceps Kickback

This exercise isolates the back of the upper arm, specifically targeting the problem area that can lead to flabby-looking upper arms.

**1** Kneel over a chair, with one arm supporting your body and one knee bent on the chair. Ensure that the elbow of the supporting arm stays slightly bent and that the knee of the leg extended to the floor is also slightly bent.

**2** With your weight in one hand, position your upper arm so it is parallel to the floor and bent at the elbow.

**3** Slowly extend the arm until it is straight, then slowly return and repeat. Do all your repetitions on one arm, then repeat on the other arm by turning around and placing your opposite leg on the chair.

**BE AWARE**
For a greater range of motion, the upper arm can be positioned with the elbow at a slightly higher angle than the shoulder.

2

3

## Triceps Dips

This exercise specifically works on toning your triceps by working both arms in one move. You will notice how quickly this muscle tones up and that this exercise will feel easier each week as the arm muscles become stronger.

**1** Sit right on the edge of a chair, with your hands next to your hips and your palms facing down.

**2** Place your feet firmly on the floor hips' width apart, with your knees bent.

**3** Lift up onto your hands and bring your hips slightly forward.

**4** Bend your elbows and lower your hips down, keeping them very close to the chair. Keep your abdominal muscles pulled in and your shoulders down.

**5** In a controlled manner, slowly push back up without locking the elbows.

**BE AWARE**
Make sure you keep your hips close to the chair to keep the focus on your triceps and not on your shoulders.

3

4

### Extended triceps dips
To make this exercise harder, simply walk your feet out a little way. Equally, to make it easier, move your feet closer in.

### Bent-Over Arm Shaper

This seated exercise will target your arms and your upper back muscles and improve your upper body flexibility and posture.

**1** Holding a weight in each hand, sit on the edge of your chair, bent over, with arms hanging down and feet slightly apart.

**2** Keep your abdominal muscles pulled in to stop your back collapsing onto your legs.

**3** Lift your arms out to the sides, up to shoulder level, squeezing your shoulder blades together.

**4** Keep the elbows slightly bent and lift only to your shoulders. Lower the arms and repeat.

### BE AWARE

To make sure you keep your arms slightly bent, imagine you are pouring water from a pitcher.

## Sitting Back Toner

This exercise uses the deltoid muscle to train your upper arms.

**1** Sit with good posture, feet hips' width apart and abdomen pulled in.

**2** Holding a weight in each hand, lift your elbows up to shoulder height, then bend them so that your wrists are by your chest and your elbows are in line with your shoulders.

**3** Using your weights, slowly squeeze both elbows behind you, maintaining the bend and keeping your elbows parallel to the floor. Hold for a second, then slowly return to the starting position.

**BE AWARE**
Aim to squeeze your shoulder blades together as you move your arms behind you.

3

## Crisscross Arms

This simple exercise tones your triceps, biceps, and chest muscles.

**1** Sit with good posture, arms extended out in front of you, palms facing each other.

**2** Cross your right arm over the left, turning your palms down along the way. Pause, then return to the starting position.

**3** Do all your repetitions on one arm, then repeat on the other arm.

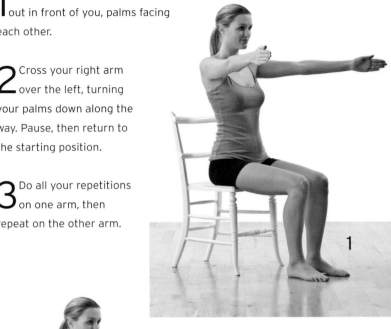

1

**BE AWARE**
Focus on keeping your abdominal muscles pulled in throughout. To make this more of a challenge, try using weights.

2

# SITTING EXERCISES

**BE AWARE**
Try to focus on just bending
the elbows and aim to
keep the shoulder joint
very still.

2

### Arms-Out Biceps Curl

This exercise tones your biceps as well
as engages your triceps because this
muscle has to stabilize the arms in the
exercise position.

**1** Sit on your chair with good upright body
posture, knees bent, and feet firmly on
the floor, slightly apart.

**2** Holding a weight in each hand, lift both
arms, fully extended, out to your sides
to shoulder height. Turn your palms so they
face upward.

**3** Keeping your abdominal muscles pulled
in, slowly bend your elbows. Aim for
your hands to reach your shoulders, hold,
then slowly straighten your arms back out.

3

## Biceps Curl

This exercise focuses on working the biceps muscle using a full range of motion.

**1** Sit leaning forward with your legs slightly spread and your left hand at the top of your left thigh.

**2** Hold a weight in your right hand and at arm's length, your elbow resting against the inside of your knee.

**3** From this position, slowly lift your arm upward to make an L-shape.

**4** With the weight at knee height, slowly lift your arm up toward your chest. Hold for a second, then lower. Slowly go all the way back to the starting position. Repeat on the other arm.

For the following floor exercises it is essential that you use a mat or a towel to exercise on. This is to protect your knees and back. As with the standing and sitting exercises, they should all be performed in a slow and controlled manner.

### Triceps Bend

This is a fantastic exercise to create tone and definition through your back arms because it isolates the triceps muscle that is found at the back of the upper arms. This muscle is toned by extending your arms straight from a bent position.

1 Lie facing up on the mat with your knees bent. Hold a weight in each hand.

2 Extend the arms straight up over your chest, palms facing in toward each other, ensuring you have a firm grip on the weights.

3 Slowly bend your elbows and lower your hands down to a few inches above your forehead, to form a 90-degree angle.

4 Squeeze the triceps muscle by slowly straightening your arms without locking out your joints.

## Kneeling Boxed Push-Up

This exercise targets lots of your upper-body and arm muscles, so it is great for toning your arms, your bust, and also for building upper-body strength. You will notice the more in shape and more toned your arms become, the stronger you will be, and you should soon be able to perform these with ease.

**1** Kneel on the mat with your knees directly under your hips. Your hands should be slightly wider than shoulders' width apart, with fingers pointing forward.

**2** Keep your body weight over your hands, abdomen pulled in tight, and your back flat. Slowly lower your body so your elbows are at a 90-degree angle.

**3** Gently push yourself back up to the starting position.

### BE AWARE
Keep your abdominal muscles pulled in to support your back and, if not using a mat, use a towel to protect your knees on the floor.

### Boxed push-up (advanced)
As you become fitter, make this exercise a little more challenging by pushing your hips forward from your knees through to your spine, so that your body is in a straight line. This means you are now lifting more of your body weight.

### Superwoman Arms

This will give tone through your shoulder and biceps, while working to improve your shoulder joint flexibility.

**1** Kneel on the mat on all fours, with your wrists directly under your shoulders and your knees under your hips on the mat. Keep your abdominal muscles contracted. Holding a small weight, lift up one arm so that it is in line with your shoulder.

**2** Now slowly bend the arm back so your elbow is then in line with your shoulder. Hold, then gently release back to a straight arm and repeat. Do all your repetitions on one arm, then repeat on the other arm.

### Back Extensions

It is important for great upper-body posture to have strong back muscles. This will help keep you strong and upright, while also giving tone through your upper arms.

**1** Lie facing down on the mat and place your fingertips by the side of your head.

**2** Contract your abdominal muscles, and keep them contracted throughout the exercise.

**3** Squeeze the back to lift the chest a little way off the floor. Hold for a second, then slowly lower back down.

## Floor Arm Lift

This is a challenging exercise, but it is
fantastic for sculpting your upper arms
because it really works your triceps.

**1** Sit on the mat with your legs straight
and held together. Place your hands,
fingertips forward, just behind your hips,
and point your toes.

**2** Pull in your abdominal muscles,
straighten your arms (hands should be
under your shoulders), and lift your hips off
the floor until your body is aligned from
shoulders to toes. Keep looking forward.

**3** Hold the position for a second, then
slowly lower to the starting position.

**BE AWARE**
To make this exercise
easier, try doing it with
your legs bent.

1

2

### Open Flyer

This floor exercise will give tone through your chest, shoulders, and arms while giving you upper-body strength and flexibility.

**1** Lie on the mat. Hold a weight in each hand over your chest, with your arms up and your palms facing each other.

**2** Keeping your elbows slightly bent, lower your arms out to the sides and down until they are level with your chest.

**3** Keep your elbows in a locked position and avoid lowering the weights too far.

**4** Squeeze your chest to bring your arms back up, as though you are hugging a tree.

**BE AWARE**
The slower you perform this exercise, the more effective it is.

## Super Chest Toner

This is a great exercise to work deep into the chest muscle, which can help to support and lift the bust muscle, as well as increase your range of flexibility through your shoulders.

**1** Lie facing up on the mat, with your knees bent and feet firmly on the floor.

**2** Holding a weight in each hand, bend your arms out to the side so they rest on the floor, elbows in line with your shoulders and bent to form an L shape.

**3** Slowly lift your arms off the floor while maintaining the bend, and aim to bring both arms to meet directly in line with your face. Hold for a couple of seconds, then slowly lower back to the floor, and repeat.

**BE AWARE**
By keeping your navel pulled down tight toward your spine, you will protect your back throughout this workout. Doing this will also tone your deepest abdominal muscles.

# COOLING DOWN

Many people dismiss cooling down after exercise as a waste of time or simply unimportant. In reality, the cooldown is just as important as the warm-up if you want to stay injury-free. While the main purpose of warming up is to prepare the body and mind for exercising, cooling down plays a different role.

The main aim of the cooldown is to promote recovery and return the body to a preexercise level and, if performed properly, to assist your body in its necessary repair process.

The cooldown will also help with "postexercise muscle soreness." It does this by allowing the muscles to repair and align themselves after the exercises. This prevents the soreness that is usually experienced the day after a workout, particularly if you have not done any exercise for a while or if you are a beginner to exercise.

Cooling down and stretching also increases your flexibility, which means you will be able to have a fuller range of movement through your joints.

## How to cooldown

Before you begin your stretches, it is a good idea to march on the spot for a couple of minutes to gently bring your heart rate and body temperature back to their preexercise state. Do this by gradually easing your march to a slow pace, then coming to a halt. Sit on the floor in preparation for the cooldown stretches.

## Postexercise Triceps Stretch

1 Sit comfortably on the mat, cross-legged and with good posture. Lift one arm above your head and drop the palm of the hand behind the head, between the shoulder blades.

2 Lift the other arm and use it to support the stretching arm on the soft, fleshy part of the upper arm or above the elbow.

3 Hold this stretch for 15 seconds. Repeat on the other arm.

2

### Postexercise Deltoid Stretch

**1** Sit comfortably on the mat, cross-legged and with good posture. Extend one arm out in front of you and cross it, still fully extended, in front of the midline of your body.

**2** Keep both shoulders facing forward. With your other hand, support the stretching arm.

**3** Hold this stretch for 15 seconds. Repeat on the other arm.

2

2

### Postexercise Chest Stretch

**1** Sit comfortably on the mat, cross-legged and with good posture. Lift your arms out to the sides and place them behind you.

**2** Keep the shoulders down as you clasp your hands together.

**3** Hold this stretch for 20 seconds.

### Postexercise Upper Back Stretch

**1** Sit comfortably on the mat, cross-legged and with good posture. Lift up your arms in front of you.

**2** Clasp your hands in front of you and imagine you are hugging a large beach ball. Feel the stretch in your back.

**3** Hold this stretch for 20 seconds.

2

Here is an easy-to-follow two-week plan. Although the plan suggests that you do a 6-minute routine each day, you can build up the amount of time you spend and the types of exercise you do. You can also mix and match the routines you choose. As you become more in shape and stronger you may feel that you can increase the number of exercises and minutes you do to a full routine. You will improve tone, flexibility, and strength.

### How to do the routines

Each daily plan has been designed to give a full workout to all the upper-body muscles. Aim to complete the number of repetitions recommended, but don't worry if you can't at first. Soon you will notice your strength and fitness improving. The routines are designed to take 6 minutes, which includes time for you to get into position and have a short rest between each exercise.

### Make the most of your workout

- Warm up and stretch before your exercises.
- Drink plenty of water to keep fully hydrated.
- Focus on keeping your abdominal muscles pulled in while exercising.
- Keep movements slow and controlled.
- When standing, keep your knees bent.
- Cooldown and stretch properly afterward.

### Day 1

Bell pull: *10-12 reps*
   p. **18**
Side shoulder raise:
   *10-12 reps* p. **21**
Shoulder press:
   *10-12 reps* p. **19**
Standing wall push-up:
   *10-12 reps* p. **19**
Triceps squeeze back:
   *15 reps* p. **16**

### Day 2

Triceps ponytail: *10 reps*
   *on each arm* p. **17**
Front arm toner:
   *10-12 reps* p. **24**
Bust lift: *20 reps* p. **29**
Upright pull: *10-12 reps* p. **20**
Bent-over arm shaper: *10-12 reps* p. **32**
Open flyer: *10-12 reps* p. **40**

## Day 3

Triceps dips: *10-12 reps* **p. 31**

Biceps curl: *10 reps on
  each arm* **p. 35**

Chest press: *10-12 reps* **p. 27**

Front raises: *10-12 reps* **p. 22**

Side shoulder raise:
  *10-12 reps* **p. 21**

Arm shaper: *10 reps on
  each arm* **p. 28**

Back extensions:
  *10-12 reps* **p. 38**

## Day 5

Front arm toner: *10-12 reps* **p. 24**

Triceps ponytail: *10 reps on each arm* **p. 17**

Chest press: *10-12 reps* **p. 27**

Superwoman arms: *10-12 reps on each
  arm* **p. 38**

Triceps dips: *10-12 reps* **p. 31**

## Day 4

Open flyer: *10-12 reps* **p. 40**

Arms-out biceps curl: *10-12 reps* **p. 34**

Triceps squeeze back: *15 reps* **p. 16**

Upright pull: *10-12 reps* **p. 20**

Shoulder press: *10-12 reps* **p. 19**

Sitting back toner: *10-12 reps* **p. 33**

## Day 6

Triceps bend: *10-12 reps* **p. 36**

Arms-out biceps curl: *10-12 reps* **p. 34**

Bust lift: *20 reps* **p. 29**

Standing long-arm palm press:
  *10-12 reps* **p. 23**

Kneeling boxed push-up: *10-12 reps* **p. 37**

Back extensions: *10-12 reps* **p. 38**

### Day 7

Triceps ponytail: *10 reps on each arm* **p. 17**

Floor arm lift: *6-8 reps* **p. 39**

Crisscross arms: *20 reps on each arm* **p. 33**

Upright pull: *10-12 reps* **p. 20**

Sitting back toner: *10-12 reps* **p. 33**

Open flyer: *10-12 reps* **p. 40**

### Day 9

Superwoman arms: *10 reps on each arm* **p. 38**

Bent-over arm shaper: *10-12 reps* **p. 32**

Arm opener: *10-12 reps* **p. 25**

Floor arm lift: *6-8 reps* **p. 39**

Super chest toner: *10-12 reps* **p. 41**

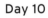

### Day 10

Bust lift: *20 reps* **p. 29**

Arm circles: *20 reps* **p. 26**

Arms-out biceps curl: *10-12 reps* **p. 34**

Boxed push-up (advanced): *8-10 reps* **p. 37**

Superwoman arms: *10 reps on each arm* **p. 38**

### Day 8

Arm shaper: *10-12 reps on each arm* **p. 28**

Side shoulder raise: *10-12 reps* **p. 21**

Bell pull: *10-12 reps* **p. 18**

Bust lift: *20 reps* **p. 29**

Kneeling boxed push-up: *8-10 reps* **p. 37**

## Day 11

Bent-over arm shaper:
*10–12 reps* **p. 32**

Triceps kickback: *10 reps
on each arm* **p. 30**

Crisscross arms: *20 reps
on each arm* **p. 33**

Open flyer: *10–12 reps* **p. 40**

Turning press: *10–12 reps* **p. 22**

## Day 13

Super chest toner: *10–12 reps*
**p. 41**

Arm circles: *20 reps* **p. 26**

Arm opener: *10–12 reps* **p. 25**

Back extensions: *10–12 reps* **p. 38**

Shoulder press: *10–12 reps* **p. 19**

## Day 12

Triceps squeeze back:
*15 reps* **p. 16**

Arms-out biceps curl:
*10–12 reps* **p. 34**

Sitting back toner:
*10–12 reps* **p. 33**

Chest press: *10–12 reps* **p. 27**

Arm shaper: *10–12 reps on
each arm* **p. 28**

## Day 14

Extended triceps dips: *10–12 reps* **p. 31**

Bust lift: *20 reps* **p. 29**

Front arm toner: *12 reps on each arm* **p. 24**

Sitting back toner: *10–12 reps* **p. 33**

Super chest toner: *10–12 reps* **p. 41**

# INDEX